Weight Reduction Through Hypnosis

Weight Reduction Through Hypnosis

Babu Moses

Library of Congress Control Number: 2009904911
ISBN: Hardcover   978-1-4415-3865-9
                Softcover   978-1-4415-3864-2

This book was printed in the United States of America.

To order additional copies of this book, contact:
Xlibris Corporation
1-888-795-4274
www.Xlibris.com
Orders@Xlibris.com
60893

1 Feb 2008

Babu Moses offers a vehicle to good health. The author describes how we can utilize our thought processes to relax our bodies and control our dietary choices. This will lead to the prevention of many illnesses and maximize one's daily functioning. Maximize your mind control and become more self-reliant then share your newly discovered power with others, as has Mr. Moses.

Timothy Mailloux, MD

Health, as defined by the World Health Organization is a combination of physical, social, and mental components. The role of the mind in determining health is very important. Many research articles have illustrated that mental health is crucial to rebuilding the individual's social and physical health. Hypnosis is a valid mechanism to assist an individual in the attainment of physical, social, and mental health. The role of medical hypnosis is documented in the literature as a positive mechanism to attain health.

This program helps the individual attain one of the most important aspects of health: weight control and weight loss, a multibillion-dollar industry. In the case of fad diets and the fad products that accompany them, most fail because the underlying issues or causes are not addressed.

This CD provides the users with techniques they can use for the rest of their lives for attaining weight loss and keeping that weight off. The self-help mechanisms described in this CD will aid the individual to take charge of his or her mental component of health which, in turn, will help the individual to increase their social interaction and physical activities.

Roger M. Nelson, PhD, FAPTA
(Fellows of the American Physical Therapy Association)
Professor, physical therapy
Lebanon Valley College
Annville, PA 17003

I have personally known Mr. Babu Moses for more than fifteen years, and he is experienced and commendable in his professional life. The work Mr. Moses has written on weight reduction is accurate; once we set our mind to lose weight, the results will occur. Losing weight is a difficult matter, and if we have the tools such as hypnosis, it can be an easier task to overcome. Congratulations, Mr. Moses, you deserve all the credit for your hard work in this area.

Lara J. Serro
Executive director
The Bristal at East Meadow

I have been acquainted with Dr. Babu Moses, who is a board-certified electromyographer and a physical therapist. He and his association have come up with a very effective way for weight reduction through hypnosis. The article he recently wrote talks about this new method. It is highly detailed and shows a step-by-step procedure on how this technique is carried out.

Dr. Babu starts out talking about the various things that tie together and contribute to who we are. He tells us what a person's emotions, self-esteem, and self-image have to do with his or her weight. If a person is compassionate, positive, and willing, then it will be easier for him or her to lose weight, as opposed to angry, frustrated, and withdrawn. Those who portray positive energy and have positive thoughts will be able to do more things and live longer lives than with negative energy. If you believe you can do something and feel good about yourself, then others will believe the same thing, and it will help you in losing a significant amount of weight.

If you imagine and visualize yourself having a great physique and act and behave in that manner, weight reduction is achieved by being motivated. When you become aware of your wrong eating habits and how it has harmed you, then you will change it using these methods.

Hypnosis offers different, better views to the mind and body. It turns the disturbed thoughts and negative self-image into something better and increases the awareness of the problem that changes the unhealthy diet and feelings. It makes you want to transform yourself in a better way and pushes you forward. Hypnosis makes you realize that overeating leads to many diseases and a faster death and offers you the alternative of facing the challenges in a constructive manner.

Relaxation, self-confidence, and a calm mind will bring out a new person. Every day when you get up, you will feel great and energetic, and so you will in the end when you reach your dream weight. When you have finally arrived at your goal weight, things will only get better. You will receive huge bouts of happiness and have great health.

I have witnessed some of his clients who have lost forty to fifty-five pounds. Hypnosis allowed them to control their emotions and focus on losing weight. As new thoughts and new behaviors emerge, self-consciousness about being overweight diminishes. After hypnosis, they could all live the life they always wanted to live.

Rasheed U. Jafar, MD
Board-certified cardiologist

Weight reduction through hypnosis is a magnificent method to lose weight; It focuses on eliminating the cause of being overweight from emotional, physical, and mental aspects. Losing weight while sleeping and waking up the next morning with a renewed spirit and mind is just amazing.

Vera Crucio
Wellness Director
The Bristol at East Meadow

This is a magnificent and powerful tool. Dr. Babu teaches one how to use mind power to succeed in our lifelong struggle. Dr. Babu also shows how we can conquer not just weight problems but other important issues of our life. Thank you for taking the time to create such an informative tool, Dr. Babu.

Winsome E. Bent, RN
Executive Director at Bristol at North Hills

Preface

There are several times that I have been asked to write a foreword or a testimonial for a published piece of work, but very few times I accepted the challenge. Indeed, it presents a challenge to thoroughly evaluate a piece of work and recommend it to thousands of people. When I was asked by Dr. Babu Moses to foreword his publication, the choice was really easy.

It is really an honor to be asked to write the foreword for this publication, an honor not only because of the caliber of the work itself but also because of the caliber of the author.

In our troubled world, a world where people feel so insecure about the future, where war and terror makes people feel insecure about their safety, where financial instability magnifies everyday stressors, we are all in need of some **relaxation**.

At a time that competition in many areas of life brings anxiety to people, a time where job security is not there anymore, where executives, workers, and students feel they may be defeated by the obstacles and problems of life, they are in need of **encouragement**.

At a time that people do not feel excited about making healthy choices, about exercising, loosing weight, quitting smoking, and creating a healthier lifestyle, they are in need of **motivation**.

Relaxation, encouragement, and motivation are leading concepts that are not only referenced in this piece of work but applied and achieved if you follow the program.

The author, Dr. Babu Moses, is not only an outstanding health care professional but also a distinguished scholar who has dedicated his life for the common good, for the good of people. He has worked very hard to produce a piece of work that can make a significant difference in people's lives. He has tremendous experience working with thousands of people and helping the majority of them to achieve the higher goals they wanted from their lives. Dr. Moses has now taken this life experience and transformed it to words and sentences creating an amazing piece of work.

I strongly recommend this publication to all those who want to achieve relaxation in their lives and to all those who are looking for encouragement, motivation, and achievement of a higher goal.

This piece of work is a gift that Dr. Moses is making to mankind!

Dimitrios Kostopoulos, PT, Ph.D., D.Sc.
Hands-On Care Physical Therapy
Hands-On Seminars (718) 707-6970

Weight Reduction Script

Dr. Babu Moses

Allow your body to get into a comfortable position as you are listening to my voice. As you are listening to my voice, you are relaxing your mind and your body from head to toe. As your mind and body become more and more relaxed, you may readjust the position of your body to become more comfortable.

Take three deep breaths. Let go all tension, all worries, all concerns from your mind. One more breath and your mind is clear as the blue sky. Imagine that you are in a whirlpool with water splashing all over you. As the warm water splashes on your neck muscles, all the tension disappears. Now the warm water splashes on your back muscles, taking away all the tension. Now water splashes on your chest and stomach, both hip knee and ankle muscles. All muscles are very relaxed. You are going deeper and deeper into a pleasant relaxation. As I start counting from one to ten, your mind is becoming more and more receptive to my suggestions. You are receiving all the beneficial suggestions both consciously and subconsciously. One, you are calm. Two, you are relaxed. Three, you are in control. Four, you believe in your abilities. You are confident that you are achieving your desirable weight. Five, you are visualizing your new body. Six, you feel happiness at the thought of your success. Seven, you are passionate about health. Eight, you are courageous to change. Nine, you are excited about your new determination. Ten, you are visualizing your new body and enjoying your success.

You are focusing and concentrating to my suggestions. Any sound other than my voice intensifies your concentration, making you highly suggestible. You are aware of unhealthy eating habits. You are responsible for the food you eat. Unhealthy eating habits are the cause of many diseases. Certain foods can slowly poison your body. Any food in excess brings the adverse effect instead of nourishing the body. They affect the health. We need food to live, to give energy, and to give us health. If you do not use the energy you get from the food, the energy stays in the body, and you gain weight. You are what you eat; thus, mind the amount you eat and the food you eat from now onward. You are thinking about your physical body and health. The extra weight burdens your heart, your lungs, and most of the organs in the body. When the heart is overloaded with work, it affects the blood vessels. These fats called cholesterol affect the arteries, clogging the blood vessels to the heart, resulting in heart attack. When they obstruct blood vessels in the brain, it results in stroke, which means half of the body is paralyzed. Blood is life, and when the blood is filled with cholesterol, the organs are affected. Fat, when deposited in the organs causes various diseases. Fats in the body contribute to diseases like cancer, high blood pressure, diabetes, and many other diseases.

As you are aware of the problems caused by overeating, from now on you are taking time to eat wisely. Think about your health before you put any food in your mouth. You are consciously asking, "Is this good for my health?" If the food is not contributing to your health, you should prefer healthier food. You should also eat the right amount. No more overeating. As soon as you are not hungry, you are totally satisfied. You do not eat more any more. You have the power over your eating habits. You have control over your food. Food is no more your weakness. Your determination to achieve your desired weight is stronger than your desire for food. Your emotional attachment to eating has disappeared. Every time you see unhealthy food, your desire is changed into achieving your desired weight. You are constantly visualizing your desired physical appearance. Your dream of attaining your desired weight reflects in your confidence, your belief in yourself. Every time you say no to fattening foods, which used to be your favorite food like steaks, bread, fast foods, sweets, salty snacks, and other junk foods, your confidence is doubles. Your belief is doubled. It is becoming easier to avoid these foods.

As you are listening to your mind more, seeking the guidance, you are more relaxed. Anger, frustration of past failures, and disappointments disappear. In the past, those emotions drove you to eat more. Anxiety, insecurity, and any stressful situation led you to eat more. Now your knowledge, your newly gained power, and your ability to deal effectively with these emotions direct you in the right path. You are enthusiastic about your commitment. You are passionate about reaching your goal. Your ideal figure is becoming a reality, motivating you to tune your mind with the body. You are eating healthier, nutritious food in small quantity. You have absolutely no desire for fattening food. You are no longer tempted to eat unhealthy food. You enjoy drinking plenty of water, eating salads, fish, chicken, turkey, and fresh fruits. The new way of eating energizes you more, satisfies you more. You are proud of yourself, enjoying a sense of well-being. You are in control of the food you eat. Food has no control over you. You are in control of your emotions. No one has the power over you and affect your emotion. Anger, fear, hostility, anxiety, and insecurity are caused by our own response. You are completely free from all the fattening food even in your thoughts. Your mind is filled with the image of your ideal physical body. You are a beautiful person. See yourself. Visualize yourself. Make the figure as clear as possible. You eat only the food that suits the new you.

You are determined. Your self-control, your willpower, your perseverance make each day easier and easier. You are energetic, vibrant, healthy, slim, trim, and attractive. You have achieved your desired weight, wearing your favorite clothes. You are happy, confident as you have more energy. You are exercising, firming up. You love the way you feel after exercising. Your strength is increasing. Your endurance is increasing. Your joy of exercising is empowering you to continue to enjoy your body more and more. The magnificent feelings of pride in achieving your desired weight and your physical appearance control your eating habits each and every day.

At the count of ten, you are emerging from this experience filled with calm, peace, and joy. One, be calm. Two, be relaxed. Three, be in control. Four, visualize your desired weight. Five, imagine your desired body. Six, be filled with confidence. Seven, be joyful about the achievement. Eight, be energized. Nine, be empowered. Ten, be wide-awake.

Weight Reduction Through Hypnosis

Babu Moses, PT, DSC, ECS. MTC, CHT (USA)

Board-certified Electromyographic Physical Therapist,
American Physical Therapist Association

You have been born in this world to enjoy living, and every day of your life is a celebration of your successful living. You are blessed with two great gifts: your mind and your body. You are responsible for using your mind and enjoying the earth's blessings through your body. As you feed your body, it responds accordingly, influencing your body size, physical energy, resistance to disease, and longevity. Your mind is consumed by dominating thoughts and responds by developing your character.

Your thoughts are the world you live in. Each and every achievement of humankind is born from creative thinking. You create your own destiny, living in heaven or hell, just by your thoughts. When you live successfully, achieving your heart's desires, your life is filled with joy, happiness, and peace. The mind creates emotional, physical, and mental productivities. Depending upon your thought process, your mind's productions can be either to your advantage or disadvantage.

Emotions like love, compassion, courage, and confidence engage your creative energy while anger, bitterness, depression, frustration, guilt, and sadness are destructive to your peace of mind. Functioning both consciously and subconsciously, your mind shapes your emotions with values that motivate you, like love, success, intimacy, security, health, comfort, power, and freedom, or values that rob your happiness, including rejection, anger, loneliness, humiliation, inferiority, failure, and guilt. Your self-esteem and self-image are the most influencing factors of the mind, developing in response to your dominant emotions and thoughts.

The only successful way of weight reduction, therefore, is through your mind power, which is enhanced by hypnosis. Weight reduction is successful and permanent only when the change happens in both the conscious and subconscious levels. It is necessary to believe in order to remove the resistance in your subconscious mind and to use your conscious mind's creative thinking to reinforce the effects of hypnosis.

Hypnosis for Health and Happiness

Hypnosis refers to the relaxed state in which you become highly responsive to suggestions. Your mind controls all the activities of your body, including your eating habits. Hypnosis enhances the power of your subconscious and conscious mind through positive suggestions. Each positive suggestion motivates the desire for weight reduction; the strong desire to lose weight is important for your success. Hypnosis has helped millions of people all over the world to reduce weight and some to achieve their dream physique. This powerful and successful method of weight reduction involves positive suggestions, removing the resistance in your subconscious mind using awareness techniques, and presleep exercises, along with hypnosis to reduce your weight and to motivate you on the exercises. It is important for you to understand the power of the mind to use thoughts, emotions, visualization, and the conditions that increase the effects. It is also important to understand who you are, what you eat, and how you want to live.

The Nutrients for Health and Happiness

Good nutrition is essential to nourish your vital organs and for physical and mental well-being. You are what you eat. A healthy diet is the foundation of health, but overeating any of the basic nutrients is harmful to your body. By choosing the healthiest of these four nutrients, water, carbohydrates, proteins, and fats, you provide your body to function at its best. The basic nutrients are water, carbohydrates, proteins, and fats, along with vitamins, minerals, and micronutrients. By choosing the proper diet, you can achieve healthy eating habits, nourishing your body with balanced nutrients.

Water is an essential nutrient for the body and forms more than two-thirds of it. It removes the waste products from microorganisms and prevents toxins from accumulating in the body. It also transports nutrients to various part of the body. Water is necessary for digestion, absorption of nutrients, circulation, and excretion. Since water is important for maintaining body temperature, it is essential to drink eight glass of water a day to ensure optimum health, reducing hunger, balancing body fluids, and quenching thirst. One glass of water shut down midnight hunger pangs for almost 100 percent of the dieters in a university study. Lack of water triggers daytime fatigue. Preliminary research indicates that eight to ten glasses of water a day can significantly ease back and joint pain for up to 80 percent of sufferers. A mere 2 percent drop in body water can trigger fuzzy short-term memory, trouble with basic math, and difficulty focusing on a computer screen. Adequate water is also known to decrease the risk of colon cancer by 45 percent, bladder cancer by 50 percent, and breast cancer by 79 percent.

Carbohydrates energize your body to function properly. They are found almost in all plants, fruits, vegetables like peas, and beans. There are two groups: simple and complex. Simple carbohydrates include fruit sugar, table sugar, and lactose sugar. Fruits are one of the richest sources of simple carbohydrates. Complex carbohydrates include sugars, fibers, and starches. Foods rich in complex carbohydrates include vegetables, whole grains, peas, and beans. Carbohydrates are major sources of blood sugar that fuels the body cells including brain and red blood cells. It is converted into glucose, and the excess glucose is stored as fats. When choosing carbohydrate-rich foods, unrefined foods such as vegetables, peas, beans, whole grain products, and fruits are best. Refined foods such as soft drinks, desserts, candy, cakes, and sugar are naturally high in simple sugars, fats, and calories. In excess, refined foods are the main cause of diabetes and hypoglycemia (low blood sugar).

Proteins are essential to provide your body with energy and are important for growth and development. They are also essential for the manufacture of hormones, antibodies, enzymes, and tissues. Protein is found in meat, poultry, fish, cheese, eggs, milk, legumes, and leafy vegetables. Since meats contain fats, soybean products, tofu, yogurt, and other soy products are healthy ways to complement the diet.

Fats are necessary for normal brain development, energy, and growth. Excessive fat intake is a major cause of obesity, high blood pressure, coronary heart disease, colon cancer, and many other diseases. The liver uses saturated fats to make cholesterol. Excessive intake of fats also increases high cholesterol. It is important not to consume more than 20 percent of fats in daily intake.

The Power of Thoughts

Thoughts are powerful, creating everything in this world. You are what you are because of your thoughts. They direct your life, create your heaven or hell, and they are your world, where you live, all the time. Your thoughts control your perceptions of the world as you live and establish your relationships with others. Since your thoughts and emotions are dependent upon each other, they also guide your eating habits. Thoughts create your character, personality, attitude, habits, and appearance. Thoughts of love, compassion, confidence, and forgiveness focus on developing a positive self-image in you. Thoughts of anger, frustration, resentment, hostility, untruthfulness, hatred, self-pity, depression, and other emotional disturbances create a negative self-image. Self-image is your concept of yourself: how much you love and respect yourself and how you develop in response to your thoughts.

Since appearance is an important factor of your self-image, your healthy eating habits contribute in developing a positive self-image. Eating the proper foods in the right amounts is a habit representing your attitude and your personality. You are responsible for any food that goes into your body. Overeating is like slowly poisoning your body and soul. Eating without conscious control may result in life-threatening diseases, especially for individuals with a family history of hypertension, diabetes, cancer, and heart disease. Since thoughts manifest your inner self in various activities, physical activities are also important to balance your calorie intake. Simple aerobic exercises like walking and jogging strengthen the muscles, increase your cardiothoracic condition, and improve your blood circulation. If your calories are not balanced by physical activities, excessive calories are converted into fats.

It is important to analyze your eating habits to understand why you eat certain foods knowing they are not healthy. If you are not happy and joyful about your life because of your eating and drinking habits, you have the power to choose to bring your eating habits under your conscious control. You can achieve your desirable, optimum weight by being responsible for your physique. If your physical appearance is not the way you desire it to be, take control of your eating habits and physical activities to achieve more in your life.

The techniques described here are simple but very effective in creating a new of way living. You already have the mind power; now these exercises increase your power, combining your body, mind, and spirit. When the change takes place in your subconscious mind, it becomes permanent and powerful. Through your thoughts, you can develop your character, personality, and quality of life, and in addition, your desirable appearance. There is never anyone like you in the whole universe.

Thoughts and Emotions

Think with feelings of happiness that you have already achieved your desirable weight. Since the mind does not differentiate between reality and imagination, if you strongly believe that you have already achieved your goal and fill your mind and body with that happiness, joy, and excitement, your mind and body accepts that new belief. That thought is your emotional pathway toward reaching your goal. When the thought is strengthened by the emotion, your mind responds with actions, and the subconscious mind absorbs the thought.

What you are today is the result of your past thoughts. The greater your desire, the stronger your imagination about how you want your dreams to come true. Vividly imagining every detail of your physical appearance and feeling the resulting emotion of that achievement opens up your subconscious mind. Since the subconscious mind accepts the imaginations as true, your thoughts, imagination, and visualization become true.

The way you are today is the result of your self-talk (internal communication), self-hypnosis (focused, repetitive thoughts), and self-image (feelings about self). What you have been thinking about yourself or imagining about your physical appearance as a result of false belief has led you to eat unhealthily. If you reflect on how and how long you have been imagining your physical appearance, you will understand the result of your thoughts.

Emotions and Diet

There is a strong relationship between a healthy diet and your emotions. The foods you consume are your pathways to health or illness. You may have consumed without paying much attention to nutritional values. When you eat foods containing more carbohydrates like rice, potato, and bread, you develop a big abdomen. It is not only the extra weight that is dangerous but also the fats surrounding the vital organs, like heart and liver, that result in heart attack or stroke. Even thin persons with extra fats in the abdomen are also at risk of these dangerous conditions.

Losing the belly fat is more important than losing weight; a large amount of visceral fats wraps the vital organs like the heart, liver, and kidneys, greatly increasing the risk of diabetes, blood pressure, heart disease, stroke, and cancer. Being overweight is a slow killer that punishes the body.

Sometimes you transfer your emotions to food without analyzing the situation. Anger, boredom, jealousy, rage, frustration, depression, and anxiety are some of the emotions that result in your unhealthy eating habits. Negative emotions are harmful to both the mind and the body, leading to eating unconsciously. I have seen that anger can stimulate chemicals, causing increased risk of heart attack; fear stimulates stress and phobia, and guilt diminishes healing energy. All these emotions contribute to eating unhealthy foods.

In this highly competitive and controlling world, it is easy to lose yourself in unhealthy living. Even though you are aware that obesity, high cholesterol, high blood pressure, and diabetes are risk factors for heart attack, you eat irresponsibly in various stressful conditions. Even Alzheimer's disease, a condition in which brain cells are killed by protein, is more common in those with high cholesterol.

Some negative emotions that influence our eating habits are anger, pride, and jealousy. Bitterness, resentment, and anger divert you from the goal of weight reduction. Analyze your part in the hurtful deed or words, then talk with the other person, directing toward forgiveness as well as repentance. Criticism about being overweight is a common reason to feel hurt. However, instead of brewing like a volcano, which leads to destruction, use creativity to change into purposeful activity.

Overcoming obstacles or adversity increases your confidence. Envy and jealously reduce your confidence and diminish your motivation for weight reduction. Thinking about the cause leads toward your overcoming the negative experience and helps to you to pursue your weight reduction.

All his life, David, a thirty-five-year-old man who was forty pounds overweight, had acted like a chicken without skin. He was angry, hostile, defensive, and aggressive at the slightest irritation. He was on disability because of his obsessive-compulsive disorder and was emotionally drained, without energy for living. After a few sessions of hypnosis, he could understand clearly that his anger was like a tempest destroying him and others in his life. Once he understood the importance of controlling his emotions, he focused on weight reduction. Now he is a man who has learnt to control both his emotions and his eating habits. He has successfully trained his mind not to be prejudiced and not to fret about small things. He has realized through awareness exercises to be self-conscious about being overweight. The extra pounds diminished as he imposed the new thoughts and a new behavior.

You need to have confidence that you will be successful in weight reduction by visualizing yourself having already attained your target weight. Confidence is the ability to believe in yourself, expecting the best and overcoming the limitations successfully. It also overcomes and confronts any feelings of self-worthlessness. Emotionally charging each word is the key to the subconscious. Unwanted weight stresses the joints, increases the heart's workload, and brings feelings of hopelessness and helplessness. When it persists, it leads to negativism, depression, and anxiety. Even though you do not eat more after gaining weight, you do not enjoy food. After eating, there is the sense of a lack of energy and preoccupation with negative thoughts. After successfully reaching your desired weight, healthy eating becomes a pleasure. Be courageous enough to change, consciously choosing the healthy way of living. Fill up your mind with youthful, energetic, and powerful thoughts.

Overeating may also reflect your attitude about others who have caused you pain, suffering, bitterness, or humiliation. Sometimes your resentment builds up, resulting in defensiveness, loneliness, insecurity, and emotional disturbances, leading you to forget about healthy eating habits. Nurturing parents may still have a tendency to overfeed you, not realizing the disadvantages of overeating.

The effective way to deal with such unresolved emotional scars is to move on with life, forgiving and forgetting totally. By repeatedly forgiving and consciously letting go of resentment, you free yourself from emotional turmoil. You have to forgive yourself for the past unhealthy eating habits. It is also important to have a strong self-image so that you are responsible for both your emotional and physical well-being.

> Adrian kept eating chocolates, ice cream, and fast food, even against medical advice. He claimed that he could not move on with his life by forgiving his ex-wife, Susan, and his best friend, Brian. Susan, his wife of five years, left Adrian to marry Brian. The agony of losing his wife to his best friend dragged him into a miserable life of unforgiving anger and hopelessness. Fortunately, before the roots of bitterness could spoil his whole self, especially his health, he responded well to hypnosis.

Power of the Unconscious Mind

Hypnosis, a state of mental and physical relaxation, is a natural altered state of consciousness that passes the conscious mind and accesses the deeper, powerful subconscious mind. In this state, there is amazing power of visualization, imagination, and suggestions, producing a real and permanent change depending upon your suggestibility, how strongly you experience the emotions associated with the suggestions, and your power to visualize and imagine vividly.

An automatic, habitual eating pattern is developed by our beliefs, values, cultures, and customs. All changes take place in the mind as mind and body function together. Physiological, emotional, and intellectual changes proceed from the mind, and the body responds accordingly. Medicines work efficiently when you firmly believe in the medicines. When you doubt and lose confidence, resistance impedes health and happiness, resulting in misery and distress. Emotions like fear, despair, anxiety, worry, depression, and mood changes create a wall of negative emotions. You need to transcend past failures, difficulties, and limitations created by your past thoughts with a new, healthy, and adventurous goal.

Setting up a new healthy habit and at times not following it gives the feeling of guilt. As your internal integrity wants to correct the situation, renewing your commitment and deciding to follow your commitments takes you back to your success. Be aware that changing inner attitudes and beliefs can change the physical appearance. You create new possibilities, emotions, and feelings by using your mental powers. Your emotions and feelings are influenced by your relationships. You have to achieve your wholeness, fullness, and completeness to appreciate the unique qualities you are empowered with.

Motivation comes in realizing your power of perseverance and persistence, but creative change occurs in an instant. Your mind is like a computer. When reprogrammed with new thoughts, actions, feelings, and emotions and reinforced with affirmative suggestions, it can achieve your desirable weight and appearance. Since emotions are also the function of the subconscious mind, the more you feel an emotion, the greater is your commitment. It is encouraging to realize how the magnitude of pain, suffering, difficulties, and troublesome experiences motivate us to change. The most driving forces are health, happiness, and success. Your mind wants you to eat wisely so that you may celebrate the joy of living.

Deep Breathing for Relaxation and Concentration

Your breathing pattern has a connection with emotions because breathing is under the influence of the subconscious, just like digestion and the functions of the heart. When you breathe consciously, paying attention to inspiration and expiration, it relaxes your mind and body. During inspiration, imagine these words: "I am taking the gift of life, filling me with positive energy." During expiration, imagine, "I am blowing out all negativity." The effective breathing that relaxes your body is the deep diaphragmatic breathing where the diaphragm, the main muscle of respiration, is used. In diaphragmatic breathing, the abdomen bulges out during inspiration and sinks in during expiration. Repeating that three or four times relaxes your body and calms your mind and then you can breathe in your usual way.

Deep breathing and associated relaxation of the body creates calmness of your conscious mind, opening up your subconscious mind. As you are thinking about these words, you are slowly drifting into deep relaxation. This relaxation induces your heightened receptivity to suggestions. As your mind is fully concentrating and focusing without distraction, new suggestions are programmed in your conscious and subconscious mind. Deep breathing during hypnosis enhances relaxation, awareness, communication within, learning, sensation, feeling, emotion, memory, and decision.

Hypnosis involves using powerful words that evoke emotions, creating a vivid imagination. You use your vivid imagination to visualize images in your mind. Visualization relaxes and takes you deeper into a hypnotic state. Positive suggestions given at this time are as seeds planted in the subconscious mind. The suggestions along with the associated feelings and emotions have great power to create changes in this hypnotic state. What the mind believes and perceives the body reflects in action and behavior.

The body is controlled by the mind; even to move the little finger, the mind thinks and orders the body to react. If the mind commands the body to relax, it is impossible for it to remain tense. Any thought, suggestion, or imagination energized with emotion is accepted in the subconscious as truth. When you imagine in your mind that you are in a beautiful place surrounded by loving people, the body also reacts as if you are there. The experience is felt in the mind, and the body responds by relaxing and loosening, without questioning whether it is reality or imagination. This is your body and mind relation, as one responds to the other through your thoughts. Most psychological sicknesses are developed in response to the dominant thoughts. The mind imagines, and the body follows.

Whenever you do any thing automatically, you are using your subconscious mind. In hypnosis, you are imagining as if you have already achieved your goal, living in that feeling and emotion, so that the subconscious accepts them as true. Again, the subconscious mind responds to the feelings and emotions without discriminating between truth and imagination. Your conscious mind behaves and acts according to those beliefs and emotions. Hypnosis is a process in which dominant thoughts and suggestions are accepted in a relaxed body and a calm, receptive mind; In short, we are who we think, imagine, and act we are.

The Power of Hypnosis

Anxiety about overeating results in emotional pain and anguish, thus increasing the chances of coronary heart disease, cancer, hypertension, and diabetes. Thoughts and feelings like failure, worthlessness, or rejection often interact, resulting in overeating unhealthy food. In fact, at times it seems being overweight is like self-punishment, bringing disturbed thoughts like selfishness and overindulgence in food. These thought patterns form a negative self-judgment, resulting in an overindulgent eating pattern. These negative thoughts lead to the formation of a negative self-image, thereby defining your self-esteem. In this state of mind, reinforcing negative thoughts leads you to disastrous eating habits. Hypnosis increases your awareness of the problem and changes the automated unhealthy eating patterns, feelings, and body sensations at a deeper level.

Hypnosis offers new experiences for the mind and the body, offering alternative views. Your mind changes according to the new information, both external and internal patterns that once interacted in a different pattern. When the suggestions reach both your conscious and subconscious mind, the conscious mind evaluates the reasons for weight reduction and focuses on taking the body to the desired state. Even though weight reduction is the goal, the negative mindset that has led to your unhealthy overeating is changed to one that encourages skillful planned action. You act and behave as if you have already lost the weight. You are joyful and excited in fulfilling your dream of achieving the perfect weight and body shape. Focusing on your specific goal at the targeted time period, you have overcome obstacles and limitations.

Hypnosis empowers the mind. You are learning to concentrate and be aware of your thoughts, emotions, and feelings. Concentration is the ability to stay focused on suggestions and visualize them with emotion. When your mind tends to wander, you bring it back to focus using your emotions and feelings. Eating is your pleasure and has become an automated habit. By consciously evaluating the nutritional value of the food, you reinforce healthy eating habits. The freedom to select and choose the food that goes into your mouth makes you the master of your destiny. You have the responsibility for your body to live longer and enjoy the relations with your loved ones.

You remember that overeating is not a pleasure because of the diseases associated with it. Your selection of food and your conscious eating change the worn paths in your mind. Such conscious and responsible eating habits lead you successfully toward your goal. When you are agitated and emotionally disturbed, relax by taking three deep breaths, remembering the words of affirmation or presleep words. You have anchored positive emotions by pressing your thumb and the fingertip which you have used to count during presleep exercise by pressing to your bed. Regular practice erases your negative images of the past. You use all these techniques and expand your thoughts and emotions. Hypnosis lifts your mood and gives you the power, energy, and skills to meet the challenges. Weight management adds more living to your life.

Hypnosis and Healthy Eating

Eating becomes automated and is reinforced by repetition as well as quantity, quality, and frequency. Analyze the food you are eating by consciously questioning in your mind, "Is this healthy or unhealthy for me?" Taking responsibility for everything that goes into your mouth brings your automated eating habits under conscious control. Your automatic way of eating is changed by imagining a new way of eating healthier food, visualizing a small quantity of right food satisfying you and drinking water with delightful thoughts. This visualization of healthier eating also involves your newly achieved body in all minute details: the youthful-looking face, muscular arms, strong legs, and flat abdomen.

After perfecting the physical appearance, visualize the confidence this body is exhibiting by maintaining an erect posture and walking with the feeling of success. Feel your new body in your mind using all the senses, smelling the fresh new body, seeing the energetic physique, hearing the praises, touching the youthful and vitality filled body, and tasting your healthy food. Focus and concentrate; make these mental images vivid and colorful. All these sensations become stronger with practice, and the body follows the mental images.

Visualization and Weight Reduction

Visualization is in a way like daydreaming but differs very much in its results. It involves picturing or running a movie in your mind of your future success as it has already been achieved. Visualization is one of the ways to reach the subconscious mind, concentrating on creating clear, bright, colorful pictures as if the goals are already achieved. When you have lost the specific weight, how happy you are! How your frustration turns to joy! How excited you are to hear the compliments! Your attitude after your success and the changes in your lifestyle are some details of your visualization. Your visualization is limitless, and you can imagine everything you want to achieve in this life.

Once successfully achieved, visualizing becomes like a movie motivating you to succeed. After visualization, the emotions become stronger and the goals become the prominent part of your life. By changing your thoughts, actions, and emotions, you create new images in the brain through visualization. You are constantly communicating with yourself by self-talk, thoughts, visualization, and emotions. Your mind perceives in images, and every positive word becomes a picture in your mind. These positive mental images are reflected in your voice, body movements, and posture. The energy and excitement amplified in your mind reaches others through your eyes, the tone of your voice, and your body language.

In visualization, the mental images motivate and increase persistence and perseverance to overcome any obstacles. Mental images that are vivid, such as success, happiness, pleasure, hope, or victory reflect your values and beliefs. Values about your appearance, health, and personality influence you to move toward your goal with confidence. For some, the main reason for weight reduction could be to avoid a heart attack, stroke, diabetes, or dangerous blood pressure—some of the illnesses caused by being overweight. Since your life is precious, maintaining physical fitness and enjoying excellent health is more valuable than any other treasures in this world. When you are in good health and in fine physical condition, there is an inner excitement about yourself; you are passionate about physical activities, desirous of achieving the impossible.

The Influence of Self-Esteem

Self-esteem is that pervasive attitude that enables you to love, to be confident and proud, and to be happy about yourself. You truly appreciate your unique qualities and love yourself. Self-esteem, often negatively affected because of being overweight, empowers you to eat responsibly and protects you from the failure of unhealthy eating habits. High self-esteem, created by a good self-image, is what you think and feel about yourself. This self-image is developed by self-talk and thoughts about yourself. Since self-image is the inner quality or how you feel about yourself, keeping physically fit increases the self-image and self-esteem. When your self-image changes, a behavioral change also takes place, and appropriate weight reduction becomes a possibility for you. Being overweight also develops the fear of criticism and can increase painful self-consciousness. Since you are communicating within yourself constantly, your communication reflects your changed new attitude.

Bobby was a thirty-year-old man without a real job, who lived on disability and suffered from chronic depression. His self-esteem was shattered by his mother who deserted him at a very young age. He could not succeed in holding a job or a relationship. When he started hypnosis for weight reduction, he was fifty-five pounds overweight. He was motivated to retrieve what he had lost, including his physical appearance. He was burning with the desire to get better. Within a short time, he changed thoroughly, gaining his confidence, his self-esteem, and his ideal weight.

The relationships with your loved ones are also very important as they play a vital role in expanding your world. They need to understand your needs so that their support and encouragement can motivate you more. Harmonious and caring relationships depend upon communicating without misunderstanding. It is good to remember you are connected to many people through emotional attachment, and living healthily is another way of demonstrating your care and responsibility to your loved ones. It is important to maintain a journal and write your emotional, physical, and spiritual changes every day. This will help you to never to go back to your old way of eating without responsibility and to set your new direction. The old way of eating was like holes in your boat, slowly sinking your boat of life.

Self-Image and Weight Reduction

Self-image is your concept of who you are, developed by becoming aware of your thoughts, emotions, and feelings about yourself. Self-image is your power while self-esteem is using that power. It is your belief about yourself developed by your assessment of how you deal with success and failure. Also developed through the opinions of others, your self-image increases when you feel good about yourself and decreases when you feel defensive, hurt, or helpless. Self-image is your right to feel good about yourself, and focusing on healthy eating habits is one way to strengthen it. Your self-image and your new eating habits depend upon each other in achieving the desired way of living. Too many negative opinions create fear, guilt, self-hate, and other emotional hurts, limiting and imprisoning your abilities. Since the self-image is developed during your early years, some of your personality traits are focused on more than others, resulting in a fragmented self-image.

> *Eva, a nineteen-year-old student, was forty-five pounds overweight. Unlike girls her age, who date and find mates, she was withdrawn, introverted, and severely depressed. Her sister, four years older, brought her for hypnosis for weight reduction. After listening to the events leading to her present condition, it was obvious that she had been abused as a little girl and was living with lots of guilt. During the self-image awareness exercises, she was frightened to see her self-image as only in parts, not the whole person. After four sessions, she managed to see herself as a whole person and then reduced her weight using weight reduction hypnosis script. Since that change takes place in the subconscious mind, she achieved a successful weight reduction.*

Since your self-image also depends upon your appearance, not feeling good about it limits your self-image. For any positive change to become permanent, self-image has to change. By removing the negative reinforcements, which hurt self-image, a new and successful life is achieved. By removing the limits you have placed in your mind and changing your self-image positively, you achieve permanent weight reduction. Deprogramming your eating habits and aiming for a healthier and happier life is achieved through hypnosis.

Your eating habits have developed in response to your emotional turmoil, hurts, and wounds. All these resistances can be removed as causes of unhealthy eating habits through hypnosis, which involves deep breathing, autosuggestion exercises, relaxation, and visualization exercises. Taking control of your unhealthy eating habits and being responsible for your eating habits is developed though hypnosis. Overeating or loss of control over your eating habits leads to your feelings of inadequacy and lack of fulfillment in life. It is self-destructive, and it robs you of health and happiness.

Subconscious Mind and Imagination

Using your energy and power through your belief system, you can expand your ability to experience and live abundantly. Because your present condition is the result of your past belief, by changing to a new, beneficial, and successful pattern, you are achieving your desired results. As you are more aware of your present status and challenge your wrong eating habits, you create a new self-image that leads toward weight reduction. All you need to do is erase the old negative image, replacing it with your new affirming words. Believe that you have already achieved your desired weight and behave so to reinforce the new thoughts until they become automatic. Whenever unhealthy thoughts come to your mind, eliminate them by visualizing the new challenging behavior. Both the conscious and the subconscious mind are involved in this process of repetition leading to success.

Thoughts of your conscious mind are the seeds planted in your subconscious mind, germinating and growing every day. If thoughts are seeds, imagination is water, and belief is soil. Imagination is stronger than belief in that it can change your belief, as water changes the soil. Because the negative status of being overweight has created negative images resulting in unhappy, destructive patterns in the mind, it is important to visualize and create new images.

Your ideal weight is achieved by focusing on realistic self-image, your present one and the one you want. You always act, feel, and behave according to your subconscious because whatever you imagine is true in the subconscious mind. Eating habits are developed by subconsciously thinking and by repetition. The subconscious mind does not differentiate between truth and imagination. The key to change is to imagine and visualize your ideal weight as if you have already achieved it and behaving so to strengthen the self-image.

Emotions and Eating

Happiness and success are derived from living a life filled with accomplishments. Weight reduction improves your self-esteem and self-image and increases your happiness and joy of living. Your thoughts and winning feelings increase your confidence, courage, belief, and faith in yourself.

Evaluating the actions you have taken and your progress in pursuit of your goal is essential to maintaining your motivation. Feel your self-esteem increase as you change your thoughts about your achievements. Your new thoughts, with a greater purpose for life, break the chains of the past. The emotion you feel as you realize your accomplishment is the guiding light toward your goal. Because your subconscious mind is open to the suggestions you are receiving, use your creative imagination, visualization, and insights to strengthen your new way of thinking. These are the functions of the right brain, and the affirmative words become meaningful in the left brain.

Through your thoughts, imagination, and visualization you have changed your belief and increased your energy and power to a healthy self-image, self-esteem, and self-confidence. Your new choice of healthy eating is increasing the years of your life. Yes, truly, you are going to live longer through this experience, reducing the chances of the diseases caused by unhealthy eating habits. You enjoy your new life, new experience, and new growth, and you increase your life force through the methods you are learning. As you free yourself from your limitations, taking the responsibility for healthy eating, you create more life filled with excitement, enthusiasm, and joy. You appreciate your abilities, and you treat yourself with respect and dignity.

Every day you exercise and physically challenge yourself. Your posture and the way you walk reflect your courage, confidence, and self-reliance. Let every step you take demonstrate your determination, and let the swing of your arm reflect your attitude. Smile and speak pleasantly with others, celebrating the new you. Use the most empowering emotion to motivate you in creating that healthy, new pathway to reflect your new attitude. By listening to the CD and reading this booklet, you reinforce a healthy way of thinking, strengthening your commitment and belief. Your attitude and behavior are reinforced continuously.

Your body is the temple of your soul, and you achieve physical fitness and your desirable weight to enjoy and celebrate your life. Even though your body has been abused by overworking, overeating, and a lack of proper exercise, your body has worked at its best under those conditions and is life-giving and nurturing. As you are successfully reaching your goal, it is only the beginning of many more successes. The once impossible has become possible by your persistence and perseverance as you have envisioned yourself and overcome your obstacles and weaknesses. You are now able to pursue other worthy purposes of your life in the same way you have dealt with your weight reduction. These days your self-image, your personality, and your concept of yourself are changing to liberate your talents and special skills. In fact, you are becoming aware of your lost talents and hidden potential to bring more joy and happiness into your life. While growing up, you ate without responsibility. Now you are maintaining healthy eating habits. All your previous limiting concepts about exercise and healthy eating are now challenged through your new self-reliance. By freeing yourself from the prison of being overweight and bringing it under your conscious control, you are opening to limitless possibilities. You are a brilliant inspiration, spreading hope and joy.

Every day is a new day, and you welcome it with renewed strength, wisdom, and power. Everyone you meet on this special day is touched by your kindness, cheerfulness, courage, and love.

As you have reached your desired weight, you look younger, and your mind is filled with youthful thoughts. You are not poisoning your body by eating the wrong foods; and you are not poisoning your mind with anger, jealousy, fear, hate, worry, or fear. Speak so that people will enjoy the beauty of your words. Smile with courage and confidence. Your presence is healing, helping, and inspiring. You are complete by achieving your dream weight, and this is health, harmony, and power.

You have succeeded in achieving your desired weight by believing in yourself and confidently moving forward and managing your emotions. This knowledge and control are adding more value to your health and happiness. You are aware that feeding the body with healthy food enriches your body, and feeding your mind with healthy thoughts enriches your mind. This is successful weight reduction. You have the power to change using the power of your mind, and this is the greatest gift in life.

In conclusion, now you are aware of deep breathing as a tool for relaxation and focus, the power of your thoughts and the gift of your visualization in achieving your ideal weight. You have the choice of alternating among the self-image enhancement script, the weight reduction hypnosis script, and the exercise-motivation hypnosis scripts, along with daytime and presleep exercise. This program is created with utmost devotion to help you achieve weight reduction in a very powerful way.

The scripts are written to achieve your goals. Physical fitness motivational script is included to explain the importance of exercises. Self-image enhancement script is given to increase awareness of the body. Daytime exercise, presleep exercises, and the weight reduction hypnosis script are more important for weight reduction program.

Daytime Exercise Script

These are mental exercises to increase your creative imagination and visualization. Performing them at least twice a day is necessary to calm the mind and body so that the subconscious absorbs your thoughts. It usually takes four to six weeks for the suggestions to become automatic.

For the first few days, you need a quiet, peaceful place without distraction. Commit yourself by focusing and concentrating on the words. Feel every word with the emotion of that word. Repeat the suggestions after relaxing the body with deep breathing.

Sit comfortably in a quiet place. Close your eyes if it is possible. Take three deep breaths, thinking you are breathing in positive power and blowing out all negative thoughts.

I am calm. I am relaxed. I am in control. I am calm. I am peaceful in my mind. The calm, secure, safe feeling is spreading all over me. I am relaxed. I let go all the tension from my body, let go all the muscles. I am relaxed. I am in control, in control of my emotions and my eating habits. I am in control. I am calm. I am relaxed, and I am in control. Every breath I take, I go deeper and deeper into a deep relaxation. All the muscles in my body are totally relaxed. I feel safe and secure. I feel the rays of comfortable sunlight spreading all over my body, gently warming up and relaxing me, totally relaxing my body. Now I am breathing in deeply. All positive thoughts are filling my mind. I am breathing out. All negative thoughts and feelings are leaving me. I breathe in positive thoughts and positive feelings. I am calm. I am relaxed. I am in control. My subconscious mind is now open to receive the beneficial suggestions.

I am happy about my commitment to reduce my weight by one to two pounds a week and lead a healthy and successful life. (Repeat three times.)

I am not going to slowly poison my body by overeating. (Repeat three times.)

I need my body to live longer, healthier. (Repeat three times.)

I am in complete control of my eating habits. I am calm. I am relaxed. I am in control. I am happier because I have achieved my desired weight, and I am healthier and younger. (Repeat three times, and open your eyes.)

Presleep Exercise

Tonight, before falling into sleep, make yourself comfortable by taking three deep breaths and letting go the tension in your body.

I am calm. I am relaxed. I am in control.

I am happier because I have achieved my desired weight, and I am healthier and younger. (Repeat twenty times.)

Every time you repeat the sentences, press the finger to the bed, starting with right-hand thumb. Keep repeating the sentences and counting by pressing the index finger. After counting five times with the right hand, repeat the counts using the left-hand fingers. After completing ten times, count with the right hand fingers until fifteen. Continue counting with the left-hand fingers and complete twenty times.

It is very important to do this exercise every night for the subconscious to be programmed with the new thoughts. If you repeat each count visualizing every word, the next day is going to be very positive to all the suggestions you have given. Since you have anchored this state of mind by pressing the finger, by pressing the finger with the thumb at any time, you experience this peaceful and empowering moment.

Self-Image Enhancement Script

Make yourself comfortable as you listen to my voice. You feel safe and secure here. As you are listening to my voice, you are relaxing your mind and your body from head to toe. As your mind and body become more and more relaxed, you may readjust the position of your body to be more comfortable.

Take three deep breaths. When breathing in, say, "I am breathing in the gift of life, filling with positive thoughts," and when breathing out, "I am letting out all the negative thoughts." Repeat it three times and then breathe in your usual way. While breathing, focus on your breathing and the way your body is positioned. Feel how you are breathing in and out. And think of the words you repeated during the deep breathing. Now focus on your body. Feel how you are lying down. Be aware of your body, the warmness of your body, the space it is occupying, its heaviness. the pressure it is creating. Consciously think about how much pressure each and every part of the body is exerting. Now focus on the position of your body. Your head, is it in the middle or turned to the side? Just feel the neck, the curve of the neck, the tension in the neck muscles. If there is any tension, press the head down on the pillow and feel the contraction of the muscles. Repeat this three times and let go the tension from the muscles. Now focus on both the shoulders, in between the shoulders, the lower back, and the sitting muscle, the back of the thighs, the calves, and the feet. Focus on the way they are and consciously think about the space they are occupying. Again, concentrate on heaviness, warmness, and position. Now, again take three deep breaths. Is there a change in the way you are breathing now? Is your chest expanding more this time? Are you breathing more than in the beginning? Now focus on the front of your body, the chest, how much it is moving up and down, to the sides. Now take one more deep breath. Is there any change in the way you are breathing now? Now focus on your abdomen, how it is rising up and down with each breath. Focus on your thighs, knees, ankles, and both feet. Is there any change in both lower extremities? Is one of them longer than the other? Is one heavier than the other? Do they feel different in any way? Now take three deep breaths and feel the difference in your breathing. Are you breathing more deeply? Does your chest expand more than before? Now close your eyes. See your image in your mind's eye. Gently press your head. Feel the tension in the neck muscles. Make each and every bone in the neck pass that pressure to the last bone in the lower back. Focus and repeat three times pressing the head and feeling the pressure on each and every bone, to the last bone in the lower back. Now without performing the movement, do it in your mind. Repeat it three times. Now perform the exercise from head down, feeling every neck bone, chest bone, and the backbone till you feel the end of the lower back.

Breathe deeply three times and see your image in your mind's eye. Is there any change in your image?

Imagine the numbers 12, 3, 6, and 9 are written on your lower back like a circle, 12 on the lumbar back bone, 6 on the sacrum. Other numbers written just like a wall clock. Now move make a circle starting from twelve to one. Repeat it five times.

Now without performing it physically, do it in your mind three times.

Now perform circles three times and feel the difference.

Now take three deep breaths. See your self-image and feel the difference.

As you practice this exercise every day, you are increasing the connection between your mind and body. Consciously performing these exercises, focusing on breathing, imagination, and movement, changes the self-image and transforms the individual.

Weight Reduction Hypnosis Script

Take three deep breaths and make yourself comfortable. As you are breathing in, think that you are taking the gift of life into you. When you are breathing out, think that you are breathing out all negative thoughts. Now breathe in your usual way and adjust yourself as you relax more. As you listen to my voice, imagine healing, comforting hands touching you body. You feel very relaxed. You let go all the tensions. These hands are now touching and gently massaging your head and your face. All the tension disappears. Now the hands massage your neck, your back muscles, taking away all the tension. Now your chest and the stomach. Now your hip, knee, and ankle muscles. Now all muscles are very relaxed. Now you are going deeper and deeper into a pleasant relaxation. As I start counting from one to twenty, you are relaxing, and your subconscious mind is becoming more and more receptive to my suggestions. You are receiving all the beneficial suggestions both consciously and subconsciously. After counting to ten, the word *deep sleep* is used. It only means that your body is very relaxed as if you are in a deep sleep, but both your conscious and unconscious mind are alert and open to the suggestions. One, you are calm. Two, you are relaxed. Three, you are in control. Four, you believe in your abilities, and you are confident that you are achieving your desirable weight. Five, you are visualizing your new body. Six, you find happiness at the thought of your success. Seven, you are passionate about health. Eight, you are courageous to change. Nine, you are excited about your new determination. Ten, you are visualizing your new body and enjoying the success. Eleven, deep sleep (continue to twenty). You are focusing and concentrating on my suggestions. Any sound other than my voice intensifies your concentration, making you become highly suggestible. You are aware of unhealthy eating habits. You are responsible for the food you eat. Unhealthy eating habits are the cause of many diseases. Certain food can slowly poison your body. Any food in excess brings the adverse effect. Instead of nourishing your body, it affects the health. You need food to live, to get energy, and to give you health. If you do not use the energy you get from the food, the energy stays in your body and you gain weight.

Since you are what you eat, the amount you eat, and the food you eat, from now on you are thinking about your physical body and health. The extra weight burdens your heart, your lungs, and most of the organs in your body. The heart is overloaded with work and stressed. Too much fat in the food affects your blood vessels. The fats called cholesterol affect the arteries, clogging the blood vessels to the heart, resulting in heart attack. When they obstruct blood vessels in the brain, they results in stroke, which means one side of the body may be paralyzed. Blood is life, and when the blood is filled with cholesterol, the organs are affected. When it is deposited in the organs, it causes various diseases. Fats in the body contribute to diseases like cancer, high blood pressure, diabetes, and many others.

As you are now aware of the problems caused by overeating, from now on you are taking time to eat wisely, thinking about your health before you put any food in your mouth. You are consciously asking, "Is this good for my health?" If the food is not contributing to your health, you prefer healthier food to that food. You are also eating the right amount, no more overeating. As soon as you are not hungry, you are totally satisfied. You do not eat more. You have power over your eating habits. You have control over the food you eat. Food is no longer your weakness. Your determination to achieve your desired weight is stronger than your desire for food. Your emotional attachment to eating has disappeared. Every time you see food, your desire is changed to achieving your desired weight. You are constantly visualizing your desired physical appearance. Your dream of attaining your desired weight is reflected in your confidence, your belief in yourself. Every time you say no to fattening foods, you have no emotional attachment to your favorite foods like steak, bread, fast foods, sweets, salty snack, sand other junk foods. Your confidence is doubled. Your belief is doubled. It is becoming easier to avoid these foods because you are healthier, vibrant, and energetic.

As you are listening to your mind more, seeking guidance, you are more relaxed. Anger, frustration over past failures, and disappointments disappear. In the past, those emotions drove you to eat more. Anxiety, insecurity, and any stressful situation led you to eat more. Now your knowledge, your newly gained power, and your ability to deal effectively with these emotions direct you in the right path. You are enthusiastic about your commitment. You are passionate about reaching your goal. Your ideal figure is becoming a reality, motivating you to tune your mind with your body. You are eating healthier, nutritious food in small quantities. You have absolutely no desire for fattening food. You are no longer tempted to eat unhealthy food. You are enjoying drinking plenty of water, eating salads, fish, chicken, turkey, and fresh fruits. The new way of eating energizes you more. It satisfies you more. You are proud of yourself and enjoying a sense of well-being. You are in control of the food you eat. Food has no control over you. You are in control of your emotions. No one has the power to affect your emotion. Anger, fear, hostility, anxiety, and insecurity are caused by your own response. You are completely free from all the fattening food, even in your thoughts. Your mind is filled with the image of your ideal physical body. You are a beautiful person. See yourself. Visualize yourself. Make the figure as clear as possible. You eat only the food that suits the new you.

You are determined. You have self-control, willpower, and perseverance to make each day easier and easier. You are energetic, vibrant, healthy, slim, trim, and attractive. You have achieved your desired weight and wear your favorite clothes. You are happy, confident as you have more energy. You are exercising, firming up. You love the way you feel after exercising. Your strength is increasing. Your endurance is increasing. Your joy in exercising is empowering you to continue to enjoy your body more and more. The magnificent feelings of pride in achieving your desired weight and physical appearance controls your eating habits each and every day.

At the count of ten, you are emerging from this experience filled with calmness, peace, and joy. One, be calm. Two, be relaxed, Three, be in control. Four, visualize your desired weight. Five, imagine your desired body. Six, be filled with confidence. Seven, be joyful about your achievement. Eight, be energized. Nine, be empowered. Ten, be wide-awake.

Physical Fitness Motivational Script

Take three deep breaths and start to let go of yourself. Relax deeper into your whole body. Imagine that you have vigorously performed a physical activity of your choice. This physical activity is relaxing your whole body, making you go deeper into a pleasant relaxation. Just adjust your body to the comfortable position you want. As you are taking deep breaths, remember that with every breath, you are filling your lungs with energy and power. The negative thoughts, stress, tension, and hurt feelings are disappearing as you breathe out. Resume your usual breathing whenever you want.

To relax more and more, you are receiving a massage to your whole body, relieving all tensions and aches. The massaging hands are magical, making you relax. My voice, my words, and the massage are relaxing you more and more. As you are continuing to relax your body, your mind is calming down, and you are focusing on relaxing more. Right now, the hands are massaging your scalp, relieving the tensions from your head. Now your face, around the eyes, nose, forehead, and the chin. Tension disappears from the face. You are now letting the relaxation spread all over your body. The magical hands are now massaging the back of the neck down to your lower back. Now you feel relieved, enjoying the relaxation, calmness, and peace. The hands are now massaging your right shoulder, elbow, wrist, and finger muscles. Now it is massaging and releasing any tension left on the right side of your body, starting from your right chest, stomach, right-side pelvis, hip, knee, ankle, and foot muscles. As the right side of your body is totally relaxed, you feel wonderful. Now the left shoulder, elbow, wrist, and finger muscles. The arm is relaxed, now the left chest, stomach, left-side pelvis, hip, knee, ankle, and foot muscles. All the muscles are now relaxed, totally relaxed, without any tension. Now your whole body is relaxed; you feel comfortable, calm, and peaceful. As you are relaxing more deeply, the person with magical fingers moves away from you, leaving you to enjoy these precious moments. As your body is relaxed, your subconscious mind is opening up for all suggestions. To open the subconscious mind more, I am counting to twenty. With every number, you are relaxing more, opening up your subconscious mind. After the tenth count, instead of the word *relaxation*, deep sleep is used. Deep sleep only means your body is totally relaxed as if you are sleeping, but both subconscious and conscious minds are alert, concentrating and focusing on the words I am saying.

Now, one, you are calm. Two, you are relaxed. Three, you are in control of your emotions and feelings. Four, you are calm, relaxed, and in control. Five, you feel peaceful. Six, you are motivated to achieve your goal. Seven, both your mind and body are totally relaxing and enjoying these moments. Eight, you are totally relaxed and comfortable. Nine, waves of relaxation are flowing from your head to your toes. Ten, you are feeling calm, relaxed, and in control. Eleven, deep sleep. Twelve, you are going deeper and deeper into deep sleep. Thirteen, deep sleep. Fourteen, deeper into deep sleep. Fifteen, deep sleep. Sixteen, deep sleep. Seventeen, deep sleep. Eighteen, deep sleep. Nineteen, deep sleep. Twenty, deep sleep. Your subconscious mind is opening up to all suggestions.

Now you feel comfortable and wonderful, peacefully using your creative imagination. You are awake, almost as if you are dreaming. All the suggestions I am giving at this time are reaching your subconscious mind, the strongest power in the world.

You are aware of the fact that you have decided, and you are committed to losing your unwanted weight and achieving your desirable physique. You have chosen to eat healthier food, nourishing your body. You are thinking, imagining, and visualizing positively to energize your mind. You are in control of your eating habits, and you are also in control of your emotions and feelings. These are the precious gifts you are giving to yourself, a healthy body and a powerful mind. As you are moving toward your goal of a slimmer, healthier, happier, more attractive, and more energetic you, you are realizing the power of your mind in changing your world. No more is the food controlling you. You are in control. No more do you eat without thinking. You think before you put the food in your mouth. Every day you nourish your body with healthy, well-balanced, energizing, low-fat, low-calorie, and low-sugar foods and enjoy the food. You are visualizing the slimmer and healthier you, even while eating. Since you have more energy, you are also focusing on exercises and physical activities.

As you experience the results of losing unwanted weight, you are motivated to be physically fit in all ways. Physical activities and exercises excite you, and you are more enthusiastic about your life. You love exercises, and your desire and commitment to have your dream figure motivate you more every day. As you imagine and visualize your ideal body, you do not procrastinate or forget your exercise regimen. Every day you feel the change: your body fat is decreasing, inches decreasing from your abdomen and waist, your muscles toughening up, and your body sculpting. You exercise regularly, enjoying health, feeling stronger, and increasing your endurance and stamina. You are almost feeling like a new human being. You feel great as you hear the praises from others. You look good, more energetic, more powerful, more confident of yourself. You have the desire to feel better, the determination to look good. You exercise regularly. You focus and concentrate on your good feelings and the benefits of exercise. Your breathing is easier and deeper. Your lungs are expanding more. More oxygen gives you more power. Your heart is accommodating more and more of the hard work, increasing your endurance and better performance. Your muscles are stronger and more flexible. Aches and pains are disappearing, and your body shape is changing.

Emotionally, you feel better and better every day. The stress and frustrations of daily life vanish. The minute you think about exercises, you feel calm, peaceful, and happy. Your fear, your doubts are gone now. You are burning with determination about health and fitness, your desirable physique. Every day you look at the progress you are making—stronger arms, powerful legs, tireless muscles, flat abdomen. As extra fat is disappearing, you admire the beauty of your flat abdomen. You are excited about the exercises and the loss of extra fat in your body. Once there was fear about your body, thinking about your genetics. Now you realize that you have more control over your physical appearance.

Since you care about your physique, you limit alcohol because of its effects on the body. You are aware that regular consumption of alcohol leads to liver problems, cancer, degenerative muscle diseases, obesity, and other addiction-related diseases. You are aware of the facts about cigarette smoking, and you avoid smoking because you value the life-giving power of oxygen. The next time you are relaxing, focus and concentrate more.

At the count of five, you will wake up from this hypnosis, and your subconscious is absorbing every thing beneficial to you. One, feel calm and relaxed. Two, realize the importance of exercises. Three, be relaxed and refreshed. Four, feel perfect in every way. Five, your eyes are open. You are fully aware and feel wonderful!

References

Gupta, A. Water. Unpublished paper. 2005.Balch JF, Balch PA.

Nutrition, Diet, and wellness. In: Prescription for Nutritional healing. 2nd ed. Garden City Park, NY: Avery Publishing Group;1997:3-5.

Maltz, M., Sommer, B. Self image: The key to your personality. In: Psycho-Cybernetics. Revised ed. New York, NY:MJF books; 2000:3-8.

Electro Physiology class notes, Rocky Mountain University of Health sciences, 1999.

www.ingramcontent.com/pod-product-compliance
Lightning Source LLC
Chambersburg PA
CBHW061229280526
45784CB00006B/2698